Breathe and Nourish

The Comprehensive Wellness Guide to Fitness and Nutrition

Table of Contents

Chapter 1. Introduction

Welcome to "Breathe and Nourish: The Comprehensive Wellness Guide to Fitness and Nutrition"! If you've been looking to take a holistic leap towards a healthier, more vibrant lifestyle, this special report is your passport to transformation. We've crafted an easy to understand and apply ensemble of the best practices, tips, and tricks that revolve around fitness and nutrition. Delve into friendly workout techniques, relish an array of nourishing recipes, and indulge in expert advice on maintaining a balanced lifestyle that leaves you thriving in a world of energy every day! Infusing joy and verdant life in every facet of being, "Breathe and Nourish" is not just a guide—it is an invitation to a wholesome lifestyle revolution which offers your well-intentioned resolutions the tangible road to discovery, energy, and radiance. Come, experience a journey that will make wellness your second nature!

Chapter 2. Breathe Right: The Power of Conscious Breathing

Embarking upon a journey of wellness starts with embracing a crucial and often overlooked element of our health: our breath. Understanding the incredible power of breathing consciously can profoundly affect our physical health, stress levels, and overall well-being. So, come along, as we explore the science, benefits, techniques, and everyday incorporation of conscious breathing.

2.1. The Science of Breathing

Breathing is natural, an automatic body function we often pay no attention to unless we're short of breath after a strenuous jog or calming ourselves during stressful situations. However, the process of breathing is a complex and integral part of our body's operation.

We inhale oxygen-rich air into our lungs, where it is absorbed into the bloodstream and transported to our cells. In exchange, carbon dioxide, a waste product from our metabolism, gets expelled when we exhale. This process, known as respiration, powers life itself. However, the way we breathe—slowly or rapidly, deeply or shallowly—can influence this process and subsequently, our well-being.

2.2. Benefits of Conscious Breathing

Mindful, or conscious breathing, involves focusing on the breath—its rhythm, depth, and overall sensation. By controlling our breath, we can positively influence our mind and body in the following ways:

1. Improved Physical Health: Deep, regular breathing can promote better blood circulation, increase the oxygenation of our blood, aid digestion, and fortify our immunity.

2. Stress Reduction: Conscious breathing is a natural antidote to stress. It can activate the body's relaxation response, triggering a state of deep rest that slows our heart rate, reduces blood pressure and cortisol levels, and instills a sense of tranquility.

3. Enhanced Mental Clarity and Focus: Deep breathing increases the supply of oxygen to the brain and stimulates the parasympathetic nervous system, promoting a state of calmness and increased attention.

4. Emotional Balance: Just like it helps us manage stress, conscious breathing can also help us navigate our emotions. It has been observed to lower symptoms in conditions like anxiety and depression.

5. Energizing Effect: Deep, conscious breathing can also energize us. Oxygen plays a vital role in energy production, and having a steady supply can help beat fatigue.

2.3. Conscious Breathing Techniques

Now that we're clear on the benefits, let's explore several conscious breathing techniques that you can incorporate into your daily routine:

2.3.1. Technique 1: Diaphragmatic Breathing

Also known as belly breathing, the focus here is to breathe deeply into your diaphragm, not shallowly into your chest.

Begin by sitting or lying down in a comfortable position. Place one hand on your chest and the other on your stomach. Breathe in slowly through your nose, allowing your stomach to rise (the hand on your belly should rise higher than the one on your chest). Exhale gently through your mouth, engaging your abdominal muscles to push out the breath while your chest remains still.

Practicing diaphragmatic breathing calms the nervous system, reduces stress and anxiety levels, and helps strengthen and increase the capacity of the lungs.

2.3.2. Technique 2: 4-7-8 Breathing

A fantastic relaxing breath, 4-7-8, is a technique that involves breathing in for 4 counts, holding the breath for 7 counts, and then exhaling for 8 counts.

To begin, sit straight and place the tip of your tongue against the ridge behind your upper front teeth, keeping it there throughout the exercise. Close your eyes and take a deep breath, exhale fully to empty the lungs, and then inhale quietly through your nose for a count of 4. Hold your breath for a count of 7. Finally, exhale audibly through your mouth for a count of 8. This constitutes one cycle. Try to complete four cycles when you first start and gradually aim to extend this to eight cycles.

The 4-7-8 breathing technique can help ease anxiety, get better sleep, manage food cravings, and control or reduce anger responses.

2.4. How to Incorporate Conscious Breathing into Your Daily Life

Incorporating conscious breathing into your daily routine does not require a monumental shift. Here are a few strategies:

1. Morning Meditation: As you wake up, instead of reaching for your smartphone, sit quietly and focus on deep, rhythmic breathing for 5-10 minutes. Breathe in energy for the day ahead, setting yourself up for a calm and focused day.

2. Breathing Breaks: Throughout the day, take mini 'breathing breaks', where you detach from your tasks and focus on mindful breathing for a few minutes—ideal during stressful moments in your workday!

3. Evening Unwind: Just as you begin to prepare for bed, practice conscious breathing as a way to unwind and signal to your body that it's time for rest.

Remember, the beauty of conscious breathing is that it's thoroughly portable and anonymous. No one needs to know that, amidst the bustle of daily living, you're actively managing your physical and mental well-being. So, start practicing, and experience the tranquility and energy conscious breathing brings onto your wellness journey.

Take note that medical or mental health advice provided here is not a substitute for professional care. It's best to consult with a healthcare provider if you have any health concerns or are considering a new health practice, especially if you have a pre-existing health condition.

Chapter 3. Nourish with Intent: Understanding the Vitality of Nutrition

Healthy eating isn't merely about rigid dietary limitations or depriving yourself of the foods you love. It's about feeling great, improving your health, and more importantly, nourishing your body to its very roots. This chapter aims to serve as a comprehensive map to guide you through the meandering paths that lead you to a healthier life.

3.1. Understanding the Basics of Nutrition

Nutrition encompasses everything you consume that fuels your body. From vitamins to minerals, proteins to carbohydrates, nutrition involves not just eating but making informed and intuitive choices about what, when, and how much we eat.

Your nutrition should ideally provide you:

- Energy, measured in kilocalories;

- Macromolecules including proteins, fats, carbohydrates for growth, repair, and energy;

- Micronutrients such as vitamins and minerals for various biological processes including immune function, bone health, fluid balance, and several other functions;

- Dietary fiber to help digestion;

- And water, the vital medium in which all these processes take place.

From maintaining healthy tissues and organs to facilitating normal growth and development, good nutrition is critical in myriad bodily functions. It is also instrumental in preventing diet-related chronic diseases like obesity, heart disease, diabetes, and cancer.

3.2. Interpreting Nutritional Information Labels

It's crucial to understand how to interpret food labels or nutritional facts panels to make wise and healthful decisions about packaged food options. These usually display values based on a 2000 calorie diet, but your personal requirement may be more or less. The values for different nutrients are expressed in grams or milligrams and as a percentage of the Daily Value (% DV).

Pay close attention to the serving size and calories. Avoid foods high in trans fats, added sugars, and sodium. Meanwhile, aim for foods rich in dietary fiber, vitamin D, calcium, iron, and potassium.

3.3. Balancing Macronutrients

Your diet needs to include a careful balance of proteins, carbohydrates, and fats – the main sources of energy for our body. The Acceptable Macronutrient Distribution Ranges (AMDR) suggested by the Institute of Medicine are:

- 45-65% of your total daily calories should come from carbohydrates;

- 20-35% should derive from fats;

- The remaining 10-35% should be proteins.

These ranges offer an ascertained balance which maintains health while providing essential nutrients.

Serene on the plate, a dietary balance of these macronutrients aids in sustainable weight management, furthers heart health, and tempers the risk of chronic diseases.

3.4. The Role of Micronutrients

Although needed in smaller quantities, micronutrients or "hidden hunger" are crucial for your health. They include the vitamins and minerals critical for neurological functions, bone health, and prevention of diseases.

Micronutrient deficiencies can cause severe health problems. To prevent this, aim for a diet diverse and abundant in fruits, vegetables, whole grains, dairy, and lean meats.

3.5. The Power of Antioxidants

Antioxidants are compounds that slow down or prevent the damage to cells caused by free radicals. They have been linked to longevity and reductions in chronic diseases like heart disease and cancer. Foods rich in antioxidants include berries, beans, apples, pecans, and artichokes.

3.6. Embracing a Holistic Diet

Consuming a wide array and assortment of foods ensures that one gets more varied nutrients. Each food group offers different vital nutrients, so it's essential to consume a mixture of each.

- Fruits and Vegetables: Packed with vitamins, minerals, and fibers, these should make up around half of your plate.

- Grains: At least half of them should be whole grains, rich in essential nutrients and fiber.

- Proteins: Incorporate a variety of protein sources, including seafood, lean meats, poultry, eggs, beans, nuts, and seeds in your diet.

- Dairy: Opt for fat-free or low-fat dairy products.

Remember, everyone's nutritional needs are different. A dietary pattern that meets your individual caloric and nutrition needs, fits your personal and cultural preferences, and is achievable and maintainable for your lifestyle is the best choice for you.

3.7. Planning Your Meals

Planning your meals is essential for creating balanced, nutritious, and varied meals. Remember the "plate method" to ensure balance - half a plate of fruits or vegetables, a quarter of protein, and a quarter of carbs.

Consider meal prepping, where you plan and prepare meals for the week ahead. This can be a great way to control portions, calorie intake, and manage mealtime rush during a busy week while maintaining variety and balance.

Remember, good nutrition doesn't come from strict dietary limitations but from a variety of nourishing, good-for-you foods. Let "Breathe and Nourish" guide you on this journey toward commendable health and exuberant energy!

Chapter 4. Fueling Fitness: The Harmony of Exercise and Food

To fully comprehend the intricate relationship between exercise and food, visualizing the human body as a well-oiled machine could serve as a fantastic analogy. Certain facets of our bodies are similar to the components of a machine. For the machine to function at its optimum, each of the constituents needs to perform in sync, and each constituent requires an appropriate form of fuel to operate smoothly. This chapter will delve deep into understanding the relation between our body, food and exercise — a harmonious blend that ultimately fuels our fitness.

4.1. Nourishment: The Cornerstone of Fitness

The bedrock of an effective workout routine lies in the nourishment our bodies receive. Our food choices directly impact our energy levels, performance, ability to recover, and ultimate fitness outcomes. Balancing our macronutrients - proteins, carbohydrates, and fats - is an essential part of this process.

Protein plays a crucial role in muscle repair, recovery and growth. It is recommended that athletes consume around 1.2 to 2 grams of protein per kilogram of body weight every day. Different types of proteins - whey, casein, soy, or plant-based - can be incorporated as per individual preference and dietary needs.

Carbohydrates are the body's primary source of energy, particularly during high-intensity workouts. Consuming enough carbohydrates ensures that your glycogen stores are high, allowing you to work out effectively and recover quicker post-exercise.

Fats help sustain long, low to moderate intensity exercises. Intake of healthy fats like avocados, nuts, seeds, fatty fish can also aid in the absorption of essential vitamins.

Remember, this doesn't mean overhauling your current nutritional profile overnight. Gradual shifts often have the most sustainable results.

4.2. Hydration: Threading the Tapestry

Water, often overlooked, forms the vital thread that weaves the tapestry of fitness together. Maintaining a balanced hydration strategy ensures the adequate functioning of our body activities. Dehydration can lead to decreased strength, endurance and can facilitate the onset of fatigue.

As a general guideline, try to drink at least 8-10 glasses of water daily. During workouts, aim to replenish fluids at regular intervals to mitigate sweat-related fluid loss.

4.3. Pre-Workout Nutrition: Filling Up the Fuel Tank

Eating before exercise provides the body much-needed energy to perform effectively. Aim for a balanced meal with carbohydrates, lean proteins, and some healthy fats. Keep the meal light and easy to digest. Examples might include a banana with a protein shake or whole-grain toast topped with almond butter and a dash of honey.

Do remember - timing is key. Ideally, aim to have this meal around 2-3 hours before your workout.

4.4. Fueling Up During Workout: Energy On The Go

For workouts lasting over 60-90 minutes, especially endurance workouts, it might be beneficial to replenish energy during the exercise. Energy drinks, carbohydrate gels, or even simple fruits can provide the quick energy boost needed.

4.5. Post-Workout Nutrition: Recovery and Repair

After a workout, the body is primed for nutrient absorption. Consuming a balanced meal within 45 minutes to one hour helps muscle recovery and replenishes glycogen stores. Aim for a 3:1 ratio of carbohydrates to protein. Some post-workout meal options could be a smoothie with fruits and protein powder, grilled chicken with quinoa and veggies, or a yogurt bowl with fresh fruits and granola.

4.6. Nutritional Supplementation: Enhancers Not Replacements

Supplements like multi-vitamins, protein powders, or energy bars can assist your food intake, but they should not replace whole foods. It's essential to approach them as "enhancers" that complement an already balanced diet, not substitutes. Always consult a healthcare professional before starting any supplement regime.

4.7. The Power of Listening to Your Body

Everyone's body responds differently to diet and exercise. Learning to listen and respond to your body's cues revolutionizes the way we exercise. When we're hungry — eat, when we're tired — rest. Respecting these cues helps us nurture a sustainable relationship with fitness.

4.8. Summing Up

Your fitness journey is not just made up of the steps you take on the treadmill or the lifts you execute in the gym; it is largely influenced by the energy choices you make in the kitchen. Harmonizing your food with your workouts helps to create a fortress of health that does wonders for your fitness journey.

Remember, you are the curator of your wellness, and understanding the harmony between exercise and food is the first step towards fueling your fitness rhapsody!

Chapter 5. Diet Deciphered: Breaking Down Myths and Building Balance

The world of nutrition can often appear as a daunting puzzle. We're bombarded with diet trends and fads, each advocating for different combinations of nutrients, making it hard to know who or what to believe. However, the key to deciphering these messages and building a balanced diet lies in understanding the foundations of nutrition.

5.1. Understanding Nutrients

No nutrient is an island. Each vitamin, mineral, and macronutrient is intricately connected to an array of bodily functions and overall wellbeing. To truly appreciate the nutrition jigsaw, you must understand the power and purpose of each nutrient.

Macronutrients mainly include proteins, carbohydrates, and fats.

- **Protein** is essential for tissue repair and immune function. Good sources include lean meats, dairy, beans, and tofu.

- **Carbohydrates** are the body's main energy source, sourced from whole grains, fruits, and vegetables.

- **Fats** are necessary for hormone production and vitamin absorption. Opt for healthy sources like avocados, fatty fish, and olive oil.

Micronutrients precisely are the vitamins and minerals required in minute quantities but vital for proper body function like Vitamin A, B-vitamins, and iron.

5.2. The Myth of "Bad Foods"

Labeling foods as "bad" or "good" is unhelpful and misleading. It constructs an unrealistic expectation that you must eat perfectly at all times. This can lead to guilt, stress, and unhealthy eating habits. Instead, consider nourishment over numbers, focusing on how food fuels and nurtures your body. If you truly enjoy a food that's considered less healthy, it's about balancing it with healthier foods and not outright abandoning it.

5.3. Fad Diets and Quick Fixes

One of the most pervasive myths is the idea of quick fixes. Fad diets promise fast and impressive weight loss, but often at a cost of your health and sanity. They are generally unsustainable and can lead to nutrient deficiencies and unhealthy eating patterns. Long-term, balanced and flexible eating patterns have the upper hand.

5.4. Eating for Energy

Food is your body's fuel, providing the energy required for daily activities. To harness this energy effectively, it is crucial to consume a balance of macronutrients. Focus on complex carbohydrates (like whole grains and vegetables) for sustained energy, pair them with protein for muscle repair and recovery, and don't overlook the importance of healthy fats for satiety.

5.5. Meal Planning and Prep

Planning your meals is a practical way to manage your dietary intake and ensures a balance of nutrients. It also makes grocery shopping easier and shrinks the odds of resorting to less healthy, convenient options.

5.6. On Dietary Supplements

Supplements are not a replacement for a balanced diet, but they can help if your diet is lacking specific nutrients. Always consult with a healthcare provider before starting a new supplement regime.

5.7. Hydration

Staying hydrated is as vital as eating well. Aim for eight glasses of water a day, or more if you are physically active.

5.8. Cultivating Mindful Eating

Mindful eating is a practice where you pay full attention to the experience of eating, noting the colors, smells, flavors, and textures. It can help combat overeating and foster a healthier relationship with food.

5.9. Intuitive Eating

A concept parallel to mindful eating, intuitive eating invites you to tune in to your body's signals for hunger, fullness, and satisfaction. It's about building an attuned connection with your body's needs and desires. This liberating practice aids you to break free from the notorious cycle of dieting and learn to trust your body again.

5.10. Balancing Act

A balanced diet honors both health and enjoyment. It is flexible, inclusive, and free from guilt. Eating is an act of self-care, not self-control. You deserve to enjoy food in a healthy, happy way without deprivation or judgment.

In conclusion, your diet should not be a math problem, varying demands of counting calories, or a perpetually swinging pendulum of guilt and indulgence. It is a multifaceted tapestry of diverse foods, tastes, and experiences that nourish you — body, mind, and, soul!

Chapter 6. Routine Reinvented: Crafting Your Personal Wellness Plan

Let's embark on the journey of creating your unique, personalized wellness plan. This comprehensive routine will not only revolutionize your day-to-day living but will also embrace the holistic vision of health incorporating physical, mental and emotional well-being.

6.1. Understanding Your Wellness Journey

Your wellness journey is unique to you. It's not about following that fancy diet endorsed by your favorite celebrity, nor about jumping onto the latest fitness bandwagon. Wellness is about understanding your body, your mindset, your habits and your lifestyle, then crafting a plan that aligns well with these aspects. Always bear in mind there's no one-size-fits-all when it comes to health and wellness.

6.2. The Five Pillars of Wellness

Your personal wellness plan will rest on five main pillars: Nutrition, Exercise, Sleep, Stress Management, and Mental Health. Each of these aspects has a critical role in not just maintaining your body's functions but in making you thrive. Let's dive into each of these areas to gain an understanding of how we can custom fit them to suit your lifestyle.

1. **Nutrition:** Everyone needs to eat, but what, when, and how you eat can make a significant impact on your wellness. The perfect

diet is the one that satiates your taste buds, meets your nutritional needs, and fits within your lifestyle constraints.

2. **Exercise:** Adopt an exercise routine you enjoy and can sustain. Whether it's dancing, swimming, yoga, or weight training, the critical emphasis should be on consistency and enjoyment.

3. **Sleep:** Adequate rest and quality sleep are fundamental for recovery and rejuvenation. Establishing a bedtime routine can significantly enhance the quality of your sleep and bolster daily productivity.

4. **Stress Management:** Chronic stress can derail your wellness journey. Incorporate stress management strategies such as mindfulness, meditation, or hobbies into your routine to maintain balance.

5. **Mental Health:** Nourishing your mind is as essential as feeding your body. Engage in activities that fuel positivity and joy while keeping mental health concerns in check.

6.3. Crafting a Personalized Nutrition Plan

To create a personalized nutrition plan, begin by determining how nutritionally balanced your current diet is. Evaluate your diet for a whole week, jotting down everything you consume, from main meals to snacks to beverages. Identify the gap areas where you need to make changes, such as including more fruits and vegetables, reducing processed foods, or drinking more water.

Work on slowly changing bad eating habits with healthier alternatives, creating a transition that is sustainable in the long term.

6.4. Developing an Enjoyable Exercise Routine

Exercise does not have to be grueling to be effective. Choose activities that you enjoy and would look forward to doing. Remember, the aim of exercising is not just weight loss or gaining muscle mass, but also about feel-good hormones, increased energy levels, and improved overall health.

Tailor your routine based on your lifestyle, preferences, and limitations. If you are unsure of where to begin, take advantage of personal trainers or fitness apps to help guide your way.

6.5. Boarding the Sleep Express

Quality sleep is as crucial as good nutrition and regular exercise. Proper sleep hygiene means establishing a bedtime ritual and sticking to it.

Try dimming the lights a few hours before bedtime, cutting off any electronic devices, and creating a calm and serene atmosphere in your bedroom. Consider options like listening to soft music, reading a book, or practicing deep breathing exercises just before bed to help signal your body that it's time to relax and sleep.

6.6. Stress-less Living

While a certain amount of stress is part of living, chronic stress can undermine our health. Incorporating stress management techniques like Yoga, Tai Chi, meditation, or engaging in enjoyable hobbies can help. It could be as simple as taking a daily walk in nature or training yourself to take slow, deep breaths when feeling overwhelmed.

6.7. Mental Fitness

Mental health is the oft-ignored aspect of personal wellness plans. Your mental state can significantly influence your physical health and vice versa. Routinely check-in with your thoughts and feelings, engage in wholesome activities that uplift your mood, and never shy away from seeking professional counseling when needed.

By integrating these practices into your daily routine in a manner that aligns with your reality, you can carve a wellness plan custom-fit to you. The key here is not merely setting health goals, but reinventing your lifestyle and daily habits, one little change at a time.

Creating your personal wellness plan is an exciting journey of self-exploration, awareness, and transformation. Embrace this process and rejoice in the multitude of benefits it brings to your overall well-being, elevating you to become the best version of yourself. Learn to listen to your body, understand your needs, and align your habits and lifestyle choices accordingly- the reward will be an enhanced state of wellness and an overall enriching life experience. Remember that wellness is not a destination, but a life-long journey. So, breathe, nourish, and thrive every single day!

Chapter 7. Mindful Eating: The Path to Holistic Health

Mindful eating is more than just a diet or weight management technique; it is a practice that helps you understand and appreciate the food you eat while tuning into your physical and emotional sensations. Incorporating mindfulness into your eating habits can help you foster a healthier relationship with food and improve your overall health.

7.1. Understanding Mindfulness

Mindfulness refers to the practice of being wholly aware of the present moment, honoring the sensations that arise without judgement. Applying mindfulness to our eating leads us to experience our meals fully. It helps us to distinguish between physical hunger and emotional hunger, and to appreciate the colors, smells, flavors, and textures of our food.

Understanding and practicing mindfulness in general is a helpful precursor to applying it to our eating habits. Here are a few simple exercises to help you begin:

1. Sit comfortably in a quiet space and close your eyes.

2. Take a moment to notice the air entering and leaving your body as you breathe.

3. As thoughts come, let them pass without judgment.

Once you become familiar with this practice, you can start applying it to your eating routine.

7.2. Preparing for Mindful Eating

Before diving into mindful eating, prepare your environment and yourself. Pick a quiet, distraction-free space for your meals. Remove digital devices to prevent mindless eating. Take several deep breaths before beginning your meal to center yourself and enhance your mindfulness.

7.3. Principles of Mindful Eating

Mindful eating revolves around the following principles:

1. Eating slowly and without distraction.

2. Listening to physical hunger cues and eating only until you're full.

3. Distinguishing between real hunger and non-hunger triggers for eating.

4. Engaging your senses by noticing colors, smells, sounds, textures, and flavors.

5. Learning to cope with guilt and anxiety about food.

6. Eating to maintain overall health and well-being.

By practicing these principles, you can form a healthier and more holistic relationship with food.

7.4. Mindful Eating Exercises

Here are some exercises to help you establish mindful eating:

1. **Eating meditation**: Begin with a small piece of fruit. Notice the color, aroma, texture, and temperature. Take a bite, and let the flavors unfold. Notice the urge to chew quickly or swallow. See if you can detect any natural impulse to reach for the next piece.

2. **Hunger-fullness scale**: Rank your hunger on a scale from 1 to 10. One signifies extreme hunger, and ten signifies overstuffed. Aim for moderate hunger (around 3) before you eat and comfortable fullness (around 7) after you have finished.

3. **Mindful meal preparation**: Engage fully in the process of cooking. Appreciate the ingredients, notice the colors, feel the textures, smell the aromas.

7.5. Overcoming Challenges in Mindful Eating

Practicing mindful eating can sometimes be challenging. Impatience, busy schedules, and deeply ingrained eating habits can prove to be hurdles. However, remember that the purpose of mindful eating is to create a balance, not to achieve perfection. Start with one meal per day, or even one bite per meal, and gradually increase your mindfulness.

7.6. Benefits of Mindful Eating

The consistent practice of mindful eating brings about several benefits:

1. Improved Digestion: Your body needs a rest-and-digest mode to process the food you eat. When you eat mindfully, you're more relaxed, which aids digestion.

2. Weight Management: By listening to your hunger cues, you're less likely to overeat, which can prevent weight gain.

3. Better Relationship with Food: You'll begin to appreciate food more and feel less anxious about eating, developing a healthier, more balanced attitude toward food.

4. Enhanced Sense of Satisfaction: By savoring each bite, you'll feel more satisfied with smaller portions.

5. Decreased Overeating: Mindful eating aids in recognizing fullness, reducing the chances of overeating.

7.7. Concluding Thoughts

Remember, mindful eating is not a diet, or about restrictions. It is about experiencing food more intensely, eating everything that you want to eat, but not eating mindlessly or out of boredom and anxiety. It is a journey to savour each morsel, to fully enjoy what you eat, and to give your body the nourishment it needs. As you embark on this journey, you can expect not only an enriched eating experience, but also improved health and wellness. Enjoy every bite, savor the journey, and here's to holistic health!

Chapter 8. Workout Wisdom: Exercise Techniques for Every Lifestyle

Exercise— an enigma to some, a lifeline to others. Whether you are an experienced workout enthusiast or a beginner looking to make lifestyle changes, this chapter will provide you with an extensive catalogue of exercise techniques tailored to suit every type of lifestyle. Strap in, as we are about to delve deep into the realm of workout wisdom.

8.1. The Fundamentals of Fitness

Before we march forward to elaborate exercise techniques, it is essential to understand some basic yet pivotal fitness principles.

1. **Consistency**: Remember, fitness is not a destination, but a journey that requires regular commitment. Try to maintain a consistent workout routine.

2. **Variety**: Engage in a variety of workouts to keep your routine fresh and your muscles challenged.

3. **Rest**: Regular rest and recovery periods are necessary for muscle growth and injury prevention.

4. **Progression**: Gradually increase the intensity, frequency, and duration of your workouts as you get stronger.

5. **Individualism**: Every body is different. What works for someone else may not work for you. Customize your workout plans according to your body's needs.

8.2. Workout Techniques for the Sedentary

If you predominantly lead a sedentary lifestyle, the transition to an active regime might appear daunting. Fear not! Starting slow and eventually building momentum is your best approach.

1. **Morning Stretches**: Begin your day with gentle stretching exercises. This can help wake up your muscles, increase flexibility, and promote a positive mind-set.

2. **Power Walking**: This low-impact activity is ideal as it doesn't put undue pressure on your joints like jogging or running.

3. **Seated Exercises**: Engage in simple movements from the comfort of your chair, such as leg lifts, arm circles, torso twists, etc.

4. **Basic Yoga Poses**: Introduction to yoga can provide both physical and mental health benefits. Start with simple asanas such as Tadasana (Mountain Pose), Vrikshasana (Tree Pose), or Savasana (Corpse Pose).

8.3. Workout Techniques for the Busy Bees

For those always on the go, finding time for a comprehensive workout can be tricky. Here's where quick, high-intensity workouts come into play.

1. **HIIT**: High-Intensity Interval Training (HIIT) alternates between high-intensity and low-intensity exercises. It's a super-efficient way to burn fat and boost metabolism in a short time period.

2. **Tabata Training**: This form of HIIT comprises four minutes of high-intensity workouts designed to push your limits.

3. **Bodyweight Exercises**: Perfect for squeezing into a lunch break or during commercials, exercises like push-ups, squats, and burpees require no equipment and little space.

4. **Cycling or Running to Work**: If possible, skip the car or public transport. Make your commute part of your daily workout routine.

8.4. Workout Techniques for the Active Agers

Age need not be a barrier to maintaining an active lifestyle. Exercise can improve mobility, flexibility, and overall health among seniors.

1. **Water Aerobics**: This low-impact exercise strengthens muscles, enhances cardiovascular health, and improves flexibility while reducing strain on the joints.

2. **Chair Yoga**: A gentle form of yoga that aids in maintaining flexibility and balance, while performed sitting on or standing using a chair for support.

3. **Strength Training**: Light strength training, using light weights or resistance bands, can help maintain muscle mass and strength.

4. **Walking Groups**: Social, interactive, and good for the heart! Involve in a community walking group to keep exercise both fun and regular.

8.5. Advanced Training Techniques

Now, for the seasoned workout enthusiasts seeking to challenge themselves further, these techniques might fuel your zeal.

1. **Pyramid Training**: Gradually increase the weight you lift while decreasing the number of reps, then reverse the order for a complete workout.

2. **Drop Sets**: After completing your set with a particular weight, immediately lower the weight and perform the same exercise until failure.

3. **Compound Movements**: Exercises like deadlifts, squats, or bench presses, which engage multiple muscle groups, can offer a challenging full-body workout.

4. **Plyometrics**: Include jump training exercises in your routine to increase power, speed, and strength.

Remember, every 'body' has a unique rhythm. Wherever you are on the wellness spectrum, this guide seeks to equip you with valuable insights, enabling a more energetic and healthier lifestyle. Embrace these techniques, find your groove, and remember — exercising is not just about looking good, it's also about feeling robust, vibrant, and invigorated. Happy exercising!

Chapter 9. Hitting the Plateau: Overcoming Fitness and Nutrition Challenges

Taking a fresh stride in your fitness and nutrition journey can be exhilarating: watching desired changes unfold, feeling your strength increase, and savoring the vibrant flavors of your nutritious meal plan. However, there comes a point—commonly known as the 'plateau'—when progress seems to stagnate. Whether physical changes have become less noticeable, or the same nutrition plan no longer satisfies your palette or nourishes your body like it used to, hitting the plateau can be disheartening. However, it's essential to understand that plateaus are a normal part of any transformation journey, indicative of your body adapting to routines and conditioning itself to changes. Overcoming these plateaus requires a systematic and enlightened approach, which we will unravel through this chapter.

9.1. Breaking the Fitness Plateau

The fitness plateau occurs when your body becomes accustomed to the exercises and intensity levels that you've been following. In other words, your body becomes efficient at managing the energy exerted during workouts.

9.1.1. Alter Your Routine

Switch up your exercise regimen every six to eight weeks. Keep your muscles guessing by introducing new elements to your routines, varying workout intensity, types, or timings. For instance, if you're accustomed to jogging, try weaving in sprints or hill runs, or consider other forms of cardio like cycling, or swimming. Cross-training can effectively challenge your muscles in different ways and provide a fresh stimulus for growth and improvement.

9.1.2. Incorporate Progressive Overload

Progressive overload entails intentionally increasing the stress placed on your muscles during workouts. This could be by increasing the weight lifted, boosting the number of sets or reps, altering the exercise tempo, or reducing rest intervals. The key to progressive overload is to make these enhancements gradually to avoid undue strain or injuries.

9.1.3. Mind Your Recovery Time

An essential yet often overlooked aspect of overcoming a fitness plateau is ensuring adequate rest and recovery. Overtraining can prove counterproductive, leading to fatigue, reduced results, and heightened injury risk. Ensure to incorporate at least one or two rest days in your weekly schedule.

9.2. Overcoming the Nutritional Plateau

Coming across a nutritional plateau signifies that our bodies have adapted to our current dietary habits. To overcome this, consider the following strategies:

9.2.1. Reevaluate Caloric Intake

As we lose weight or gain muscle, our body's caloric needs change. Consider consulting a professional to assess your current needs and adjust your macro and micronutrient intake correspondingly.

9.2.2. Concentrate on Whole Foods

Rather than sticking to a monotonous diet that limits food groups, focus on whole foods rich in nutrients. Incorporating a wide variety of fruits, vegetables, whole grains, lean proteins, healthy fats can provide the necessary vitamins, minerals, and fibre.

9.2.3. Stay Hydrated

Often underestimated, hydration plays a pivotal role in breaking nutrition plateaus. Keeping your body optimally hydrated aids digestion, metabolism, and nutrient absorption.

9.3. Emphasizing on Mental Wellness

Last but not least, mentally embracing the plateau is just as crucial in overcoming it. Practice patience and maintain a positive mindset. Understanding that achieving fitness and nutrition goals is a personal journey that takes time and effort, rather than a race, can pave the way to eventual success.

9.3.1. Harness the Power of Mindfulness

Embrace mindfulness techniques like meditation and focused breathing to reduce stress, enhance concentration, increase body awareness, and ultimately, foster a more profound connection between your body, food, and physical activity.

9.3.2. Cultivate a Growth Mindset

A growth mindset implies embracing challenges as opportunities for learning rather than obstacles. Seeing plateaus as signs of your body's adaptability can help you explore creative solutions, leading to improved resilience and sustained progress towards your wellness goals.

In summary, don't let hitting the plateau deter your fitness and nutrition journey. Instead, see it as an opportunity to evolve your practices, reassess your goals, and further understand your body's reactions and adaptability. Equipped with these strategies, you can successfully embrace and overcome the fitness and nutrition challenges, making wellness an intrinsic part of your lifestyle.

Chapter 10. The Kitchen Corner: Wholesome Recipes for a Healthy Life

Eating is one of the life's profound pleasures, yet we often take for granted the impact of what we eat on our health. To embark on a journey towards wellness, you need to make a conscious choice to nourish your body with nutrient-dense foods that your taste buds will love. Welcome to a palette full of colors, an aroma of freshly plucked spices, and a whirlwind trip around nutritious, wholesome food that will add to your life, and not just to your waistline.

10.1. The Art of Meal Planning

The first step on your road to healthful eating is planning your meals. Too often, our busy lifestyles push us to take shortcuts, resulting in fast food, quick snacks, and frozen meals. But meal planning offers a healthier and more satisfying alternative. Here are some tips to successfully execute meal planning.

- Understand Your Dietary Needs: Every person is unique and so are their dietary needs. Understanding what your body needs is the first step in meal planning. If you have specific dietary restrictions or needs, factor them into your plan. Experts suggest that a balanced meal includes proteins, carbohydrates, and healthy fats along with vitamins and minerals.

- Plan in Advance: The best time to plan for the upcoming week is the weekend. This way you have ample time to think of creative and nutritious dishes.

- Prepare a Shopping List: Based on your meal plan, prepare your shopping list. This will ensure you buy only what you need, reducing impulse purchases.

- Batch Cooking and Portion Control: Cook in larger quantities to save time and effort. You can refrigerate these meals and have them through the week. Make sure when serving your meals you're considering portion sizes, it isn't just about what you eat, but also how much.

10.2. Exploring Nutrient-Rich Ingredients

Our bodies need a mix of different food groups to function optimally. But how do we know which foods offer the best nutritional benefits? Here's a breakdown of some of the nutrient-rich ingredients we should aim to include in our diets.

- Proteins: Lean meats, seafood, eggs, legumes, and dairy products.
- Carbohydrates: Whole grains, beans, fruits, and vegetables.
- Healthy Fats: Avocado, nuts, seeds, olive oil, and oily fish.
- Vitamins and Minerals: A mix of fruits and vegetables will aid in achieving your daily requirements.

10.3. Flavorful Recipes That Fuel You

Healthy doesn't have to be bland or boring. Here are a few easy recipes that promise a burst of flavors and wholesome nutrition.

10.3.1. Nutty Avocado Quinoa Salad

Ingredients: - 1 cup cooked quinoa - 1 ripe avocado - Half cup cherry tomatoes - Quarter cup chopped almonds - Lemon juice - Olive oil - Salt and Pepper to taste

Steps: 1. Mix cooked quinoa, sliced avocado, cherry tomatoes, and almonds in a bowl. 2. In a separate small bowl, mix lemon juice, olive oil, salt, and pepper to make the dressing. 3. Pour the dressing over the salad and toss gently to combine.

10.3.2. Rainbow Stir-fry

Ingredients: - 1 yellow bell pepper - 1 red bell pepper - 1 orange bell pepper - 1 green bell pepper - 1 onion - 300 grams tofu - 2 tablespoons soy sauce - Olive oil - Salt and pepper

Steps: 1. Sauté the tofu in olive oil until it turns golden-brown. 2. Add the onions and sauté until translucent. 3. Add all the bell peppers and stir fry. 4. Mix in the soy sauce and let it cook for a couple of minutes. 5. Season with salt and pepper.

These mouth-watering recipes, rich in nutrients and textures, can make your journey towards more wholesome food a delightful experience.

10.4. Balancing Your Plate

One key to achieving maximum nutrition is balancing your plate. However, it doesn't mean packing it with just salads or proteins. Aim to include

- Half the plate with veggies,

- One-quarter with lean protein,

- One-quarter with whole grains or starchy vegetables,

- Plus a serving of fruit and dairy.

10.5. Mindful Eating

While what we eat forms the crux of the journey, mindful eating forms an equally crucial part. Pause at meal times, polish off distractions, appreciate your food, eat slowly, and listen to your body's cues.

Embarking onto a wholesome lifestyle through the right nutrition doesn't have to be a mammoth task. The conscious endeavor to choose and prepare nutrient-filled food becomes a habit over time. And when wellness becomes a habit, every day is a step towards a healthier, better life. So let's head into the Kitchen Corner afresh, with renewed energy and enthusiasm for the betterment of our bodies, minds, and souls. Your wellness journey begins here. Happy Cooking!

Chapter 11. Recharge, Reset, Revitalize: Embracing Optimal Wellness and Recovery

Practicing optimal wellness and recovery are integral aspects of maintaining a healthy and balanced lifestyle. Born of a fine blend of self-care, self-awareness, regular activity, and healthy eating, they pave the path to physical, emotional, and mental vitality. In the quest for wellness, each one of us follows a unique journey, narrating a tale of personal progress and self-discovery.

11.1. A Symphony of Sleep

Remember, every wellness journey starts somewhere and often, it's in the slumber of sleep, that nocturnal necessity that too often simmers on the back burner of our priorities. But sleep is a crucial component of wellness, a revitalizing retreat that helps our bodies recover, reset, and recharge.

Quality sleep rejuvenates the mind, body, and soul, boosting cognitive function and emotional well-being. It facilitates physical recovery after a grueling workout session, knitting together the damage caused by the day's physical activities. Moreover, sleep fortifies our fortress of immunity and abets good heart health. Aiming for seven to nine hours of sleep each night ensures sufficient time for our bodies to undergo these reparative processes.

However, understand the true essence of sleep would require a deeper dive into your nightly patterns. Track your sleep and ensure that you're not just sleeping long, restless hours, but also reaching the restorative REM (Rapid Eye Movement) stage. Techniques like sleep meditation, maintaining a darker and cooler bedroom, and adhering to a consistent sleep schedule can bolster quality sleep.

11.2. Nature Nurtures

Upon rising, it's time to greet the day anew, armed with nourishment and nature. Spending time amidst nature has myriad benefits. It aids in reducing stress, boosts mood, and improves mental well-being. Just a brief walk in the park or observing the tree outside your window can be a delightfully effective way to commence your day.

Incorporate time in the outdoors into your daily wellness routines. Try a jog in the park, an outdoor yoga class, or even a lunch break at your favorite outdoor spot. As little as fifteen minutes of sun exposure per day is enough to boost your body's Vitamin D production - an essential nutrient that helps maintain strong bones and an agile immune system.

11.3. Food: Fuel for the Body

As we circumspectly circulate between our daily tasks, our body demands its dues in the form of food. Our meals play a pivotal role in providing the energy needed for physical and cognitive functions. Consuming meals rich in fruits, vegetables, whole grains, lean proteins, and healthy fats fosters overall well-being and primes your body for recovery and revitalization.

Of equal importance is water, our body's most essential nutrient. Carrying nutrients to our cells and helping discard waste, water is the lifeblood of our bodies. Aim to drink at least eight glasses of water a day, but remember—this figure can change based on your activity level, size, and even the weather.

11.4. Decoding Exercise

Exercise is a powerful tool aiding wellness, impacting not just physical health, but mental and emotional too. Whether it's a well-dedicated workout regimen or simple routines like walking to work, taking the stairs, or doing chores, it's all about keeping the body in motion.

Find the physical activity that truly resonates with your lifestyle and preferences. This could be anything from yoga, pilates, weightlifting, running, dancing, or swimming. Regular exercise not just simulates your metabolism and promotes better sleep, but can also enhance your mood and mental wellness. Exercise is an irreplaceable pillar of a healthy lifestyle, and it's essential to find a regimen you enjoy to maintain consistency.

Rest and recovery are also integral to any exercise program. Devote days to lighter activities or complete rest to allow your body to heal from rigorous workout sessions. Stretching, foam rolling, or yoga can serve as excellent recovery activities.

11.5. Embracing Mindfulness

Refining your vision inwards, it's now time to discuss the heart of wellness: mindfulness. In today's hectic world, nurturing mental calm can seem like a daunting challenge. But the answer lies within us, in the tranquil realms of our mind.

Mindfulness is all about being present in the moment, actively engaging with your senses, and acknowledging your thoughts and feelings without judgment. Regular practice of mindfulness, like meditation, enhances mental clarity, reduces stress, and promotes a sense of peace.

11.6. In Conclusion: The Balance of Being

Optimal wellness lies in the harmony of physical, emotional, and mental health. It implies recognizing and respecting our body's necessities and limits, establishing a sleep routine that ensures quality rest, eating a balanced diet, engaging in regular physical activity, and setting time aside for rejuvenation and relaxation. Remember, wellness is not a destination—it's a journey. Step by step, through the mindful nurturing of body, mind, and soul, we can unlock the potential to live our best, most vibrant lives. Recharge, reset, revitalize—you are but a decision away from embracing this potent triad of wellness.

www.ingramcontent.com/pod-product-compliance
Lightning Source LLC
Chambersburg PA
CBHW070742260726
48660CB00007B/2942